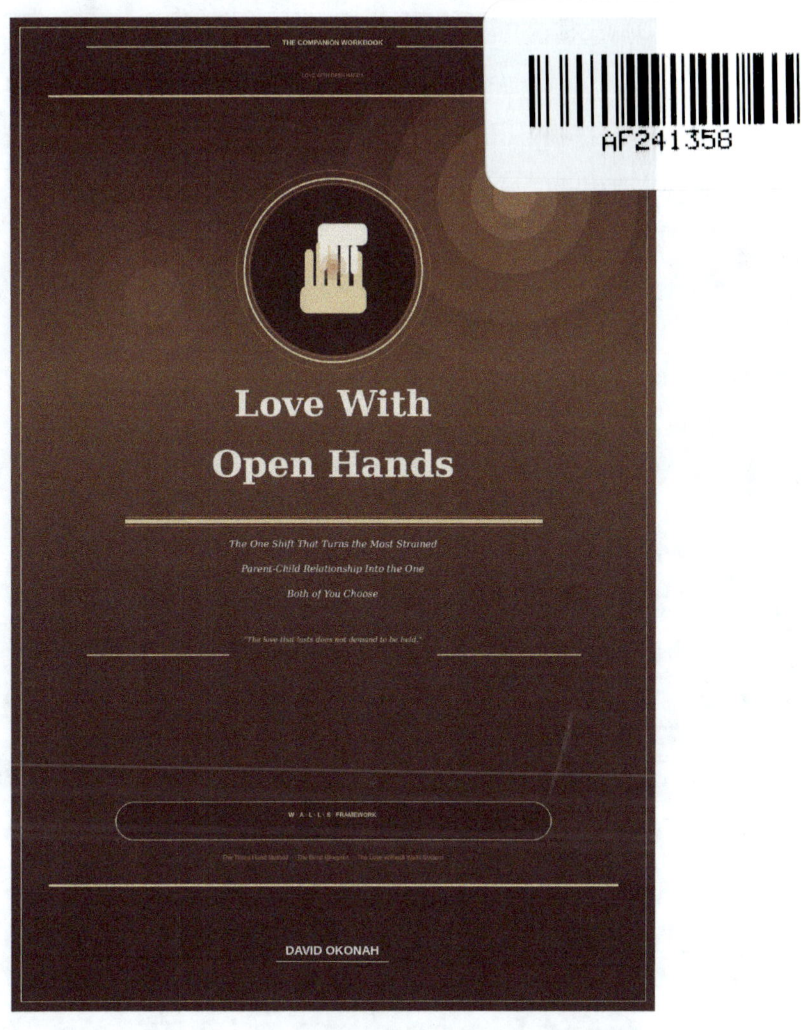

Your Name:

Date I Began:

> *"The love that lasts in any relationship is always the love that does not demand to be held."*

How to Use This Workbook

This workbook is your companion for Love With Open Hands by David Okonah. Work through it alongside the book — one chapter at a time, in sequence — though every exercise also stands alone whenever you need it.

There is only one rule: honesty over performance. Write what is true for you, not what you think you should feel. The discomfort you encounter is not a sign that something is wrong — it is evidence that something important is being seen, perhaps for the very first time.

What You Will Find Here

- Reflection exercises for every chapter of Love With Open Hands
- The complete Fear Audit — your personalised map of the patterns you are here to change
- The Three-Hand Method daily tracker — 14 days of real-time practice
- The Evidence File — your running record of your child's capability
- The Deliberate Step Back weekly practice — 6 weeks
- The Five Open Question practice cards
- The Repair Conversation framework and drafting space
- The Partner Alignment Conversation guide
- The Identity Reclamation four-week practice
- The Consistency Protocol — daily, weekly, and monthly
- The Legacy Letter — 20 writing lines and prompts
- The WALLS Quick Reference Card

A note before you begin

You are not here because you failed. You are here because the relationship matters enough to fight for. Everything in this workbook serves one destination: the day your child picks up the phone and calls you — not because they have to, but because they want to.

PART ONE: UNMASKING

Chapters 1 – 5 | Seeing the Walls

Before anything can change, you must first see — clearly, honestly, and without judgment — the patterns that have been driving the distance between you and your child. Part One is not about blame. It is about illumination.

Chapter 1: The Grip That Feels Like Love

> *"Anxiety disguised as love is not experienced as love by the child."*

Opening Reflection

Something brought you to this book. Name it here — not the polished version, but the honest one.

What brought me to this book:

The Fear-or-Care Diagnostic

Think of the last time you intervened in your child's life. Write it below, then apply the one question that changes everything.

The intervention I am thinking of:

The Diagnostic Question
"If I were not afraid right now, would I still do this?"

My honest answer:

What this tells me about my pattern:

Key Takeaway

The exhaustion and growing distance are not signs of failure. In your own words, what is the pattern you are beginning to name?

Chapter 2: The Walls We Inherited

"The walls were built by love shaped by fear, passed down through generations."

The Wall Origin Story

Answer these questions slowly. There are no wrong answers here — only honest ones.

Who first taught me that love means holding on?

What did I learn to fear about releasing someone I love?

In what ways am I parenting the way I was parented — even though I promised I wouldn't?

What pattern do I most want to end with me — so my child doesn't carry it forward?

The Generational Gift

"The cycle I am choosing to end is

and the gift I am choosing to give instead is

____

and my child will feel the difference because

____

Chapter 3: The Hidden Grief Nobody Talks About

> *"Grief that is named can be moved through. Grief that is buried drives every controlling behaviour."*

The Grief Naming Practice

Name each specific loss below. Not to dwell in it — but to honour it. What is named can finally be released.

I am grieving...

The closeness of:

____

The version of my child who:

____

The family as it once was:

____

The version of myself before I was this afraid:

____

What I most need to hear about this grief right now:

____

What I am ready to release:

How my child has been affected by this unprocessed grief:

Chapter 4: The Cost You Haven't Fully Added Up

> *"Guilt says: I did something that needs to change. Shame says: I am something that cannot change. This book works with guilt. It dismantles shame."*

The Cost Inventory

This is not a list of failures. It is an honest foundation from which genuine change is built.

What fear-driven parenting has cost my relationship with my child	What it has cost me personally

Guilt vs. Shame

> **GUILT:** *"I did something that needs to change."* This is fuel. Use it.
> **SHAME:** *"I am something that cannot change."* This is a lie. Release it.

The guilt I am converting into fuel today:

The shame story I am choosing to release:

My forward-facing commitment ("Starting from where I am today, I will..."):

Chapter 5: A Journey, a Map, and a Compass

> *"You are not lost. There is a map, a compass, and a proven path."*

The Love Without Walls System — Overview

THE WALLS FRAMEWORK

Witness · **A**cknowledge · **L**oosen · **L**isten · **S**oar

Place a checkmark next to the stage you believe you are currently in:

- ☐ W — Witness: I am beginning to see my patterns clearly
- ☐ A — Acknowledge: I am owning the full cost of those patterns
- ☐ L — Loosen: I am actively practising letting go in real time
- ☐ L — Listen: I am rebuilding the bridge through genuine curiosity
- ☐ S — Soar: I am living the relationship I built toward

The Three-Hand Method — Introduction

✊ Closed Hand	👐 Open Hand	✋ Guiding Hand
Control	*Trust*	*Mentor*

Which hand do I reach for most often right now?

What I most hope this journey gives me:

What I am most afraid of as I begin:

PART TWO: REWIRING

Chapters 6 – 11 | The WALLS Framework in Action

Part Two is where the WALLS Framework becomes a lived practice. Each chapter corresponds directly to one stage of the journey. Work through them in sequence — each stage builds on the one before it, and together they constitute the six-week Love Without Walls System.

Chapter 6: Five Walls, Five Doorways

> *"The WALLS Framework is not a philosophy. It is a map with doorways — and every doorway opens in sequence."*

The 30-Day Connection Reset — Orientation

The 30-Day Connection Reset replaces one controlling behaviour per week with a specific trust-building alternative. It runs alongside the five WALLS stages and takes no more than ten minutes per day. Before you begin, identify your starting point.

My starting commitment:

The one controlling behaviour I am replacing first:

____

The trust-building alternative I will practise instead:

____

The person who will hold me accountable:

____

(W) Witness

"See your walls clearly, compassionately, and for the very first time."

Chapter 7: See It Clearly

THE FULL FEAR AUDIT

Take your time. This is the single most important exercise in this workbook.

List your ten most frequent parenting interventions. Apply the diagnostic question to each. Name the fear beneath it.

#	My parenting intervention	Without fear, would I still do this? (Y/N)	The real fear beneath it
1			
2			
3			
4			
5			
6			
7			
8			
9			
10			

Three-Hand Identification

Looking at your Fear Audit, which hand governs most of your daily parenting interactions right now?

What I discovered about myself in this audit:

The pattern I can now see most clearly:

(A) Acknowledge

"Own it completely — on your child, your relationship, and yourself."

Chapter 8: Own It Completely

The Relationship Deep Dive

The specific moments with my child I most wish I could do differently:

The distance I can see now that I was contributing to:

What I believe my child feels when I reach for the Closed Hand:

The Partner Alignment Assessment

Answer honestly. This is private — no one else needs to see this page.

Where my co-parent / partner and I disagree most on parenting approach:

How that disagreement shows up in our home:

One thing I could say to invite them into this journey — without blame:

My Forward-Facing Declaration

"I acknowledge that

I accept responsibility for my part. Starting today, I choose to

The person I am becoming — for my child and for myself — is

(L) Loosen

"Release the grip — one deliberate, courageous act of trust at a time."

Chapter 9: Release the Grip

The Three-Hand Method — 14-Day Daily Tracker

For each high-stakes interaction, note which hand you reached for first and which you chose.

Day	Situation (brief)	Hand reached for	Hand I chose	How it felt
Day 1				
Day 2				
Day 3				
Day 4				
Day 5				
Day 6				
Day 7				
Day 8				
Day 9				
Day 10				
Day 11				
Day 12				
Day 13				
Day 14				

The Deliberate Step Back — 6-Week Practice

Each week, choose one situation from your Fear Audit. Consciously choose not to intervene. Record what happens.

Wk	Situation I stepped back from	What I feared would happen	What actually happened	What the gap tells me

The Evidence File

Record every time your child handled a difficult situation without your involvement. Read this file when the fear says they cannot manage without you.

Date	What my child handled without me	What it shows me about them

(L) Listen

"Rebuild the bridge through genuine curiosity and the radical act of hearing without agenda."

Chapter 10: Hear What They're Actually Saying

The Five Open Questions — Practice Cards

Practise one question per day. Record what you noticed.

Question 1: *"What was the best part of your day?"*
Low stakes, no agenda — opens the door without pressure.
What I noticed when I used this:

Question 2: *"What are you thinking about doing?"*
Positions your child as the decision-maker. Signals trust.
What I noticed when I used this:

Question 3: *"How did that feel for you?"*
Invites emotional honesty without requiring it.
What I noticed when I used this:

Question 4: *"What do you think you'll do?"*
Transfers agency explicitly and warmly.

What I noticed when I used this:

Question 5: *"Tell me more about that."*
Three words. The most powerful invitation available to you.
What I noticed when I used this:

The Repair Conversation Framework

The Three Things You Need to Communicate

1. *"I see what has been happening between us."*
2. *"I am working on changing my part in it."*
3. *"I am not asking you to respond. I am showing you something different."*

My Repair Conversation in my own words:

The moment and place I will initiate it:

What happened after (record this after the conversation):

The Consistency Protocol — Setup

- ☐ I will complete my daily 3-question check-in at this time each day:
- ☐ I will complete my weekly review on this day each week:
- ☐ I will share my weekly review with this person for accountability:
- ☐ I will complete my monthly WALLS assessment on this date each month:

(S) Soar

"Step into the relationship you were always building toward — and discover who you are inside it."

Chapter 11: Step Into the Life You Were Building Toward

The Identity Reclamation Practice — Four Weeks

What did I love before I was this child's parent?

What have I always wanted to try but deferred because the timing was never right?

What would I do if no one needed anything from me for an afternoon?

My one thing:

My protected one hour per week:

What I notice about myself — and the relationship — when I honour it:

My Flourish Markers

Define the specific, emotionally meaningful moments that will tell you the transformation is real.

The voluntary contact that would mean everything:

The conversation that would tell me we have arrived:

The moment I would know I am at peace:

The version of myself I am becoming — in my own words:

PART THREE: FLOURISHING

Chapters 12 – 18 | Sustaining the Open Hand

Part Three is where the transformation takes root in the real world — through the hard seasons, the resistant child, the co-parenting tension, and the ongoing work of becoming who you always meant to be.

Chapter 12: When Nothing Seems to Be Working

> *"Consistency in the absence of visible reward is the single most powerful signal you can send to a child who has learned not to trust that change is real."*

The Rupture Recovery Tool

When you fall back into old patterns — and you will, at least once — use these three steps instead of making the relapse evidence of failure.

Step 1: Name it without drama. "I reached for the Closed Hand."

Step 2: Identify the specific fear that triggered it.

Step 3: Choose one open-handed response in the next 24 hours to re-establish the pattern.

My most recent relapse moment:

____

The fear that triggered it:

____

My re-establishing response in the next 24 hours:

____

What this setback teaches me about my pattern:

____

Chapter 13: The Co-Parent Conversation

> *"The parent who brings their partner into this journey multiplies the transformation's reach into every relationship the family contains."*

Partner Alignment Conversation Guide

The Shared Observation: *"I've been noticing something about how our anxiety shows up in how we parent…"*

The Personal Ownership: *"I'm working on my part in it. I'm not asking you to agree with everything…"*

The Joint Invitation: *"I think if we could get on the same page — even partially — it would change things for all of us."*

How I will open this conversation with my partner:

What I anticipate their concern will be — and how I will receive it:

The one thing we can agree on right now, even if we disagree on everything else:

After the conversation — what shifted:

Chapter 14: Loving the Adult Child You Didn't Expect

> *"There is no age at which this work becomes irrelevant. The adult child who has been pulling away is not gone — they are waiting."*

The specific distance I am navigating with my adult child right now:

The Repair Conversation adapted for our adult relationship — what I need to say:

One open-handed act I can offer this week with no agenda attached:

What I believe they are waiting to see from me before they trust the change is real:

Chapter 15: The Teenager Who Won't Talk to You

> *"The resistant teenager is not proof that the framework doesn't work. They are proof that the parent's previous approach has been deeply felt."*

The specific hostility or withdrawal I am currently experiencing:

What the resistance might be telling me about how deeply my previous approach was felt:

The open-handed response I will offer consistently for the next 30 days, regardless of their reaction:

My 30-day open-handed commitment:
Every day for the next 30 days, regardless of how my child responds, I will:

I will measure success not by their response but by whether I held the Open Hand.

Chapter 16: Reclaiming the Parent You Always Meant to Be

> *"The parent who rediscovers who they are outside the intensive parenting role becomes, organically and inevitably, the parent their child finds most worth returning to."*

The Legacy Vision

How do I want to be remembered by my child, in their own words?

____

What does it mean to love my child in a way that left them free?

____

What am I modelling for my child about what it looks like to release fear and choose trust?

____

My Identity Declaration

> *"I am more than my child's parent. I am also:*
>
>
>
> ____
>
> *And that fullness makes me a better parent — not despite itself, but because of it."*

Chapter 17: The Consistency Protocol

> *"Insight without structure fades under the pressure of daily life. Daily practice rewires the pattern."*

Daily Check-In (5 minutes)

Each evening, answer these three questions:

1. Which hand did I reach for most today?
2. What was the moment I am most proud of?
3. What is the one thing I will do differently tomorrow?

Weekly Review Checklist (20 minutes)

- ☐ Review my daily check-ins from the past week
- ☐ Add at least one new entry to my Evidence File
- ☐ Complete this week's Deliberate Step Back reflection
- ☐ Identify my next step up the anxiety scale for next week
- ☐ Note one thing that is measurably shifting in the relationship
- ☐ Share my progress with my accountability partner

Monthly WALLS Assessment (60 minutes)

Which WALLS stage am I currently in?

____

What is measurably different compared with one month ago?

____

What practice is landing most powerfully?

What has my child done this month that belongs in the Evidence File?

What do I need more of in the next 30 days?

Chapter 18: The Relationship You Were Always Building Toward

> *"The relationship on the other side of open-handed love is not a repaired version of what existed before. It is something entirely new."*

My Flourish Vision

Paint the relationship you are building toward — in specific, warm, vivid detail. Not a fantasy. A credible, earned, entirely attainable future.

What the voluntary phone call looks, feels, and sounds like:

____

What the Sunday dinner chosen freely feels like:

____

What the adult friendship I am building toward looks like:

____

What I am doing with my own life in this next chapter:

____

THE LEGACY LETTER

Not to be sent. To be kept. The clearest evidence of who you chose to become.

This letter is not for your child to read right now. It is for you — as evidence, in your own handwriting, of the parent you have chosen to become. Write it when you feel ready.

Let these three questions guide what you write: Who have I become through this journey? What is the relationship I am building toward? What does the love I am offering now look like?

Date: _______________________

Dear ____________________,

With open hands,

Appendix: The Love Without Walls Quick Reference

THE THREE-HAND METHOD

Step 1 — Name the Hand: "Which hand am I reaching for right now?"

Step 2 — Check the Driver: "Is this coming from love or from fear?"

Step 3 — Choose the Hand: "Which hand does my child need from me right now?"

THE WALLS FRAMEWORK

W — Witness: See your patterns clearly, compassionately, for the first time.

A — Acknowledge: Own the cost — on your child, your relationship, and yourself.

L — Loosen: Release the grip, one deliberate act of trust at a time.

L — Listen: Rebuild the bridge through genuine, agenda-free curiosity.

S — Soar: Step into the relationship you were always building toward.

"The love that lasts in any relationship is always the love that does not demand to be held."
— David Okonah, Love With Open Hands

DAVID OKONAH
Love With Open Hands